This fine book by Felicia Mitchell is, strangely, Audrey McClary Mitchell. Audrey rests in Beaufort Cemetery, ___ g father and brother, but her voice is recorded, considered, mingled with her daughter's own as surely as if she were sitting beside her in the present moment of each poem. It's a book in large part about the art of listening, about the complex way memory is born and gathered and protected, a book about honoring people like Audrey whose language has become "alzheimerspeak"—a language that the impatient find unintelligible, but this poet hears as if it were lyric.
—**Joyce Dyer**, author of *In a Tangled Wood: An Alzheimer's Journey*

Through the poems in *A Mother Speaks, a Daughter Listens*, Felicia Mitchell evokes the tender and complicated emotions of accompanying a parent through dementia. Her words are compassionate, but not pitying; sad, but not despairing; familiar, but not flippant. In reflecting on her mother's dementia and death, Mitchell shares with an honesty and insight that will resonate with others who share that experience, and that can guide us all toward greater understanding and care.
—**Rev. Joanna Harader**, author of *Expecting Emmanuel*

Felicia Mitchell's bright-shining collection *A Mother Speaks, A Daughter Listens* invites us into these aching spaces and the fey-like language between mother and daughter, the two of them being "two pieces of the same puzzle." Mitchell honors not only her mother but the last, trying journey many of us must undertake. In these pages, we are not lost but blessedly found: in story, in clasped hands, in giving voice. It is certain we carry nothing out of this world, wrapped/rapt only in the beckoning light of remembrance.
—**Linda Parsons**, author of *Candescent: Poems*

I like the scope of Felicia Mitchell's book and admire her talent. It's difficult putting words together that make sense of dementia. It's a problem with language. *A Mother Speaks, A Daughter Listens* uses poetry to sketch out the space between mother and daughter. It is a lullaby sung from mother to child and back again the other way around.
—**Richard Spiegel**, The Waterways Project of Ten Penny Players, Inc.

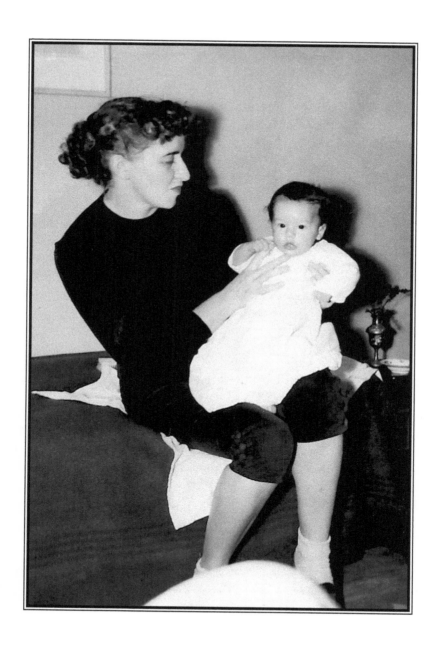

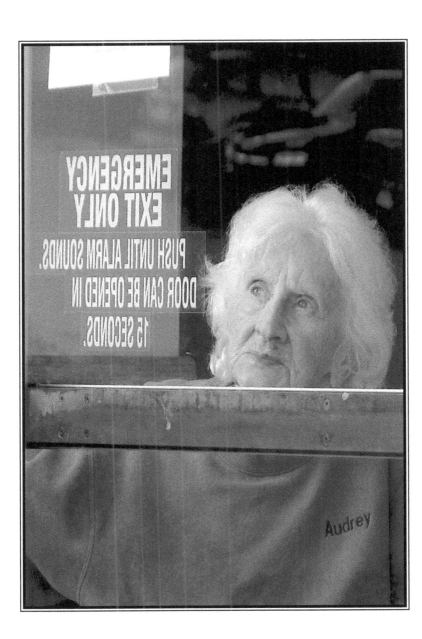

A Mother Speaks,
A Daughter Listens

A MOTHER SPEAKS,
A DAUGHTER LISTENS

JOURNEYING TOGETHER THROUGH DEMENTIA

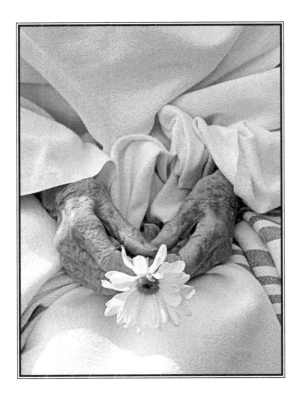

Felicia Mitchell

Wising Up Press

Wising Up Press
P.O. Box 2122
Decatur, GA 30031-2122
www.universaltable.org

ISBN: 978-1-7376940-2-1

Catalogue-in-Publication data is on file with the Library of Congress.
LCCN: 2022941055

In Memory of Audrey McClary Mitchell

CONTENTS

MOTHER'S DAY

The wind was blowing
so very hard.
The flowers nodded
in the yard.

A small young girl
with dirty bare feet
picked some flowers
and found a seat.

She was making a basket
in a child-like way.
It was for her mother,
on Mother's Day.

1969

I

remember all our stories

MEMORIES OF CHARLESTON

Audrey told her husband she remembered a ditch.
She also remembered a car and chickens.
And a calico cat she protected from the chickens
that scratched in the front yard of a big house
across from a fenced cemetery where Spanish moss
made shadows into ghosts in the early evenings.
Audrey also remembered a well in the backyard
where a woman poured water over her head
and into her thirsty mouth one hot barefoot afternoon
when all she wore was a slip to slip outside to play
while everyone else in the house napped through the heat.
And how she stayed outside until her slip and hair dried
so she would not have to tell anybody about the ghost
that came out in broad daylight to play with her
until her family woke up and called her in to supper.

My Mother's Speech Impediment

After South Carolina, in Philadelphia,
my mother would take speech lessons
to erase the Gullah words and syntax
that interrupted her sentences—
as if her mouth were some *tabula*
capable of becoming *rasa*.
                          It did not work:
her teachers shook their heads
and circled the spelling errors
that followed her syllables like shadows.
Mama knew they thought she was
just some *po buckra* off the farm,
but she knew better.

PHOTO OF A DEBUTANTE, WINNSBORO COTILLION

But Audrey looks happier in another photo,
three babies under three, dirty socks strewn on the floor,
and coal in a bucket to feed a potbellied stove.
The books on the table in this other photo
are the only tidy thing in the whole house
because the children cannot reach them, not yet.

I learned to write copying letters from these books
the way my mother learned to love, by loving our father,
my scribbles indelible as red lipstick in an old photo
of a young woman in a white, white lacy lace dress
about to step across a threshold to dance.
This woman was a woman who would wear purple
and carry African violets on her wedding day,
who would go home with her husband, my father,
to a rented bedroom in somebody else's house
until they had to move, the first time,
and then again, baby after baby,
never settling for less than happy-ever-after.
Oh, how the two of them loved to dance.

INTIMATION ODE

My brother fed me my bottle,
lying next to me in his diaper
with me in mine, so young.
We were so young
we did not need words
other than eyes and sighs,
but one day we talked.
We talked in a language
invented by angels
and understood by only us
and perhaps God,
the God who stood over us
the day our mother baptized us,
herself, far outside the city limits
where our concrete house
was as holy as the Vatican
to our father, excommunicated
for marrying our mother
and having these children
who talked like angels
while their daddy worked and worked
and their mama, pregnant again,
fed coal to a potbellied stove.
What did we say to each other?
I think we talked about that time
before we were born,
a time that hovered outside the window
like a flying saucer
only a few could believe in.
But our parents did.
They believed in flying saucers
and babies and metaphysics
and living on next to nothing
as if it was everything,
everything in the whole wide holy world.

WATEREE SWAMP

I remember how we left Mama
on a bedspread at the edge of the swamp,
nine months pregnant, with fried chicken to eat
and a shotgun to protect her from bears,
Daddy said, "bears" meaning "danger."

And she would have shot the gun too,
at a bear or a man or a renegade duck,
at anything that threatened her
or the child swimming inside her
while the other children and her husband
navigated a boat around cypress stumps
and looked for reflections in the water.

I remember that afternoon as easily
as I remember all our stories
and hold them as close as that shotgun
Mama held, or us, ready to pull them out
when I need them to protect me
from the idea that one day, someday,
nobody will know we left Mama
on a bedspread at the edge of a swamp,
nine months pregnant, eating fried chicken,
while her family disappeared into black water.

FIRST DATE

The bell buzzed through the house
like a cosmic alarm clock
waking me up from adolescence.
I do remember that but not what I wore
or how I fixed my hair that afternoon
or if my face was broken out in pimples.
I only recall rounding the bend in the stairs
after holding my breath for thirty seconds
to calm myself to meet this boy's gaze,
this boy who wanted to fall in love with me,
and seeing instead my mother at the front door.
At 54, she looked pretty good in a bathing suit.
"What's your sign?" she asked my date,
as he walked into the house that afternoon,
storing up her analysis to report on later
when he told her he was a Scorpio.
After more dates than I would count,
my mother did my boyfriend's horoscope,
summarizing: "Bad pennies always turn up."

MAMA

I had to hunt her down,
run through hospital halls
to find her pacing.

"Mama."

"He's calling you," I said,
reeling from the sound
of my brother's voice.

"Mama."

When he died,
his hand still held hers.
She had to pull it off.

Later she told me
we should not have been there:

You come into this world alone.

STILL LIFE WITH PEACHES AND CUCUMBER

Joe Belton's peaches hang heavy and ripe
right outside the house where his wife is dying.
Marie sits by the window, her wig off in this heat,
and talks about her daughters coming for Christmas,
with their husbands and children, her grandchildren.
"She still has her appetite," my mother says later,
as we drive back to Columbia laden with peaches.
I know: I saw her eat a cucumber from the Paschals' garden,
peel and all, each bite already a memory before she swallowed.
In Blythewood, everybody's garden grows.

A HALF OF A SCARF

In her uncle's well-worn sea chest,
with sweaters and her sister's schoolwork
from 1928, her son's last report card,
a strand of glass pearls her husband gave her,
and two hand-knitted shawls
made by a first cousin once removed,
is a half of a scarf from her mother.
"This is all I have left of my mother's,"
Mama says, handling it like a lock of hair
or a piece of clothing somebody special touched.
Standing next to half of a cherry table
from her father's side of the family,
she shows me the half of the scarf
that even in its best days could not have been
more than sixteen inches long.
Perhaps it was from Lerner's on Main Street,
where my grandmother liked to shop,
a fact my mother told me in passing one afternoon
when the two of us were walking downtown.
However my grandmother came by it,
it was the sort of scarf you would tuck in a collar
or a pocket, barely enough silk to matter.
Still, it is the sort of heirloom whose history
my mother does not want me to forget,
even if she never tells me the whole story
only half of her mother's story, the happy half.

AUDREY'S MEMORY

You know, I want to go to Charleston.
And that cute boy.
Before I sent into then,
we have a beautiful house there.
After Daddy and everything.
It was a very good place.
It didn't bother me.
He was so visitble,
he draw a beautiful build.
We just wonling.
Right by the water,
very beautiful water by the water.
And Brownie, she said, "Well, just do it."
And we all dived!
I liked sunsing.
We had everything.
Money.
Charleston.
I used to stare there.
They had a good time.
Two dead.
Had the same thing in it.
Right from the water.
We had a beautiful house, but he died.
It was a big, big, big house, and was so beautiful.
Where we did.
Oh, I loved it.
I can't get out and go.
But to see it.

II

why things so complicated

1990

Dear Felicia,

John and I are delighted
over your great news. Do you realize
some people my age
are great grand parents!

Happy happy thoughts—
good for babies.

Love, Mama

1994

Dear Felicia,

Love the cooler days—
sky is so blue, & clouds.

Brownie called—
leaves Mon. to go to Isabelle's, Leslie's & Graeme's.

Kitty & Nancy left Wed.
Joe is doing fine.
He had a bladder infection
which made recovery slower.
He said Walter came by
& Aunt Mary is better than she's been in 2 years—
knows some of them.

She was kept on drugs
at the nursing home
Walter said & now she is free of all that she is fine.

They give them pills
to keep them quiet & less trouble—

a shame.

Love, Mama.

1999

Dear Gail,

Your flower a beautiful pink azalea.
It was a beautiful day in Beaufort,
National Cemetery, cool & blue skies.

We had a bagpipe playing before & afterwards,
he played "Amazing Grace."

John was of 12 children,
so lots of family—mine, so many dead—

John so ill so long.
He had a lot wrong with him.
We had 45 years
after marrying 11 days after we met.
There is love at first sight.

Sincerely,

Audrey E. Mitchell

LOVE, MAMA

Dear Felicia—
At last I got up to a great rain—
been so long for a real rain!
I keep water like in the kitchen or bath
& haul it out to put on flowers.
This sand dries out so fast.
I have a lot of leaves in the flowers out front—
need to work into dirt also.
I looked at the K-Mart ticket
& one type on sale 1.33 (was 1.99)
& these two still on 1.99—
after this I'll take my look before I leave—
so many in the line that day.

FEBRUARY 10, 2000

Can you believe 75
will be here today?
I always remember
how it was so nice & warm
Feb. 17th, 1954.
I didn't even take a jacket
& after everything & night time
was still warm.
Your note came.
Thank you.

* * *

Don't understand why things
so complicated
when it should be don simple—
legal jargon (?) too much words—help—
nothing simple.

* * *

Hope this doesn't fall apart—
a rotton place along porch
has two baby birds yelling,
all I can see some grass—
up by the roof.

CHRISTMAS CARD

Jan. 27, 2003

Dear Felicia—

I did write & when I look-
ed it—too much wrong!
I saw a part of the paper—
& was a long thing & didn't go thru it—
but went back.

I'm still washing ect.
& want to fix my face & dress,
maybe I can walk a little—
the cat is on my bed again—
hate to move her out—
to cute. She called me when she stopped
& went in.

2003

At last I saw Smyth Chapel—is Smyth a E?
The Dr. from where you are his name Smythe.
He talked a lot the last Dr. I saw—
only time he had to talk—
I told him where he lived there
& moved to college here.

Nice person—
he told me not to walk anywhere home—
6 weeks at home—
& I had to work—
a year was a whole time after all he did!
A year be all to go!

I went to Dr. Baldwin yesterday—
always a long time—
had new papers—
lots I couldn't see the first at seeing to much—
I asked the girl I didn't see it to well—
so got her to do some—didn't large & smown.

Was almost 45 waiting.
I told my Dr. I need a new one—

well—
my Dr. told me he'd tell you one—
good ect.
All done right with a lady did it all—
Said I was in good still all fine he said.

*U*PDATE

Graeme is going up town
& will pick up my lost!
which isn't—
will get it—

I'll call first,
he will pick it up.

Yesterday on the street
waiting for bus to Rosewood
& then to Kilbourne
now will get 2 times in a 60 places there.

I was so cold
with just my pink around me.

MARCH 1, 3004

Last week it was bad
all most of it!
Today it is 70/53 and all the week
will be ever one 77/57.

The sunflower ones you sent are March-June.
I've go to get it up a lot.
I've been doing back at the grapes
needed cutting back—large of it—been cutting out some.

Still trees from next place—
Some fell & I cut the out—

I tried to take it us & get out but too large.

I cut it up & took up out—
Still I have come out—
homes always had large of them—
we had large ones every one.

Have to do a lot in the front—
will begin now—

thankyou sent—

LETTER TO GRANDSON, 2004

to Guy

Cup! 29.
20 for you—
Love Audrey

III

what it is

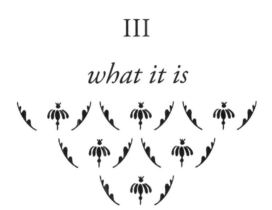

ROUND AND ROUND

I took my toddler to Sims Park
one day I felt overwhelmed
by a simple family visit.
I wanted to leave South Carolina,
our visit lasting too long,
a blizzard blocking the road home.
Sitting on the bench as my son played,
I thought of my mother's cancer
and chemotherapy treatments
I would not understand
until I went through my own.
I thought of my father,
his Parkinson's Disease
starting to show more signs.
I thought of my mother,
her dementia emergent even then.
Both of my parents were overwhelmed,
as much as I was overwhelmed,
but they had each other—
and they had their children.

Now and then, my young son looked over,
making sure I was still on the bench,
his guardian there in an urban park
where I too had once played.
When he saw me burst into tears
the day I felt overwhelmed,
he ran over and took me by the hand
to drag me onto the playground.
With his two-year-old arms,
my son spun me on the merry-go-round
until I was laughing again,
like him, my life as open to wonder
as the road to Virginia was to melting snow.

MY FATHER FAILS MY MOTHER (AGAIN)

When my father's mind begins to age,
the genius in him giving way to some confusion,
my mother starts to test him in small ways.
Overhearing her asking him what day my brother died,
as if she herself would ever forget,
I cringe because she has told me he is losing numbers.
The time he could not tell her how much an apple was,
if six apples were in a pound, is still her cross to bear.

"The sixteenth," my father assures her, wrong.

Just hearing his answer is enough to break my heart.
Knowing he is failing my mother's tests is worse:
it is enough to make my blood run hot and cold.
If I were my father's wife, I would ask different questions.

BALLROOM DANCING

When my mother accepts a dance
with an octogenarian at a wedding reception,
her arthritis takes wings
and flies out of the room
like funereal doves set free.
For minutes, her soul soars too,
reunited with the spirit of her youth
that made her belle of all balls
and got her a bit part in a B movie
where she just had to glide by.

But here came my father,
she complains to me on the phone later,
huffing and puffing, irate,
in such a jealous rage she thought she would die
right there in the American Legion.
She was so embarrassed, she recounts,
when he pulled her off the dance floor.

"He has it in his head I slipped away once,"
she explains, "when we lived in Sumter."
His story: She was gone a half hour,
and I was born nine months later.

For months after the wedding reception,
my father torments my mother, who torments me.
For years, she reminds me of this false memory,
my introduction to a Parkinson's delusion
an introduction to the magic of the genome.
Then she forgets what she told me repeatedly
and tells me that I am delusional when I mention it,
this twist in the story an introduction to her dementia
before I know exactly what dementia is.

Years later, both parents gone, their battle with them,
I will seek to learn with certitude that I am their child.

The Decision

Perhaps some people would question
how I let my mother decide
to let my father leave this world,
to pull one feeding tube and not try another,
the day she decided to let him go.
I held his medical power of attorney,
something offered years before
when my mother said to my father,
in words that would not make sense to me
until after he had passed away,
"My mind is not what it used to be."
Perhaps some would tell me I, not my mother,
should have been at that table of doctors
who listened to her when she said,
"I know death when I see it."
I believed her when she told me, though,
recounting how the decision was made
in the face of my father's body shutting down.
"One doctor did not agree," she said.
"I could see it in the way he left the room."
But the others in the meeting agreed it was time,
time to let Mr. Mitchell go ahead and go.

Perhaps some people would tell me even today
I should have exercised my own right to choose,
to delay the inevitable death of my father,
but what difference would that have made?
Mama was right, and as much as I had hovered,
watching every move she made with my father—
sometimes whispering behind her back—
this was a decision she had to think she could make.

Slop

How can I mop up after my own mother in the produce section of the grocery store when she has an accident and calls out "Boy!" It's easier to hide behind a shelf of watermelons than it is to apologize to that man for this woman who is no longer in her right mind. Should I explain that she calls me Charles? That her husband is often her father? And sometimes not anything makes much sense. Perhaps I could pretend my name is Boyd and her teeth are looser than usual today. "Okay, Mama, I'm here, Boyd's here, right here!" I could yell, so he could hear, but I don't look like Boyd. I look more like Felicia or, it's true, Miss Felicia. I look like my mother's daughter, my own superior airs worn like a shabby sweater bought once upon a time in just the right shop. And even she would look at me as if I were crazy if I decided to change my name in the produce section. Suddenly I would be the one condemned as delusional, locked up in the mind of a child taught all the wrong words in a whole other century—in a whole other country, my own. There's nothing to do but watch him slide and fall on a word that is lying there like the blood of his ancestors on some linoleum he was supposed to be mopping up. Or maybe he thinks she was excited to see the tomatoes. Maybe it's normal to yell out "Boy!" when they're so red. "She always grows Better Boy," I could say, nodding at them. "Those Better Boy bushes always yield the very best crop." Just like these tomatoes here, I could say, buying five pounds to make up for my mother's word that is still lying there, slop on the linoleum floor between that Black man and me.

AT THE S&S CAFETERIA

The woman at the next table
wants her mother to use her right hand.
"Use your right hand, Mother," she instructs,
shifting the fork from one side to the other
while green peas spill into rice like punctuation marks.
Mother, seated in a wheelchair, does as she is told,
moving food to mouth without uttering a word.

The woman at my table, my mother, eats her turnip greens
and comments on the macaroni and cheese.
She says the same thing about her food each time.
Soon she will ask for a bag for her pecan pie
so she can take it out and eat it later.

What I do at times like these is eat my slice of sweet potato pie.
It's sweet as memories spilling from Mama's mouth,
stories that get mixed up between bites of greens
and cheese that could be cooked a little longer.
I listen to every word my mother says
and watch her watch the woman spilling peas.

WHEN IS SUMMER?

When is summer?
Before you know it,
summer will be here
wagging its tail behind it.
Colorful green ideas will sleep
in the front yard,
where all winter brown leaves
drape themselves
across the roots of flowers you planted.
Yes, you!
The flowers will bloom too,
red and pink and yellow.
When is red?
Red is when months bloom
caterpillars crawling across the yard
and colorful red ideas play like kittens.
You will see the spider-like flower.
It will not bite you.
It is safe to touch.
When is summer?
Don't worry, it will come
the day after tomorrow
but before today.
Remember the time the butterfly bush
grew taller than the house?
Its colorful yellow blossoms dance
to your summerless winter
even as we speak.

THE TRICKS WE PLAY

I part my hair in the middle.
Sunday, I put on a pretty dress
and pull my hair into a ponytail.
My mother loves my shoes.
I sip green tea while she smiles.
Monday, I wear my hair
the way I did in high school,
some of it pulled back
into a flower-shaped barrette.
I buy a bottle of Wind Song.
Tuesday, I wear an old ring
my mother gave me, pink coral,
something I picked out and she bought.
Wednesday, I try to fit into a dress
I bought thirty years before,
its embroidered mirrors
reflecting a lifetime of change.
I buy kefir and decide to give up sugar.
I stand in front of hair dye at the drugstore.
Sunflower gold or honey blond?
Or should I buy curlers?
Thursday, I wear Mary Janes again.
My mother loves my shoes.
I love pomegranate seeds and salmon.
Friday is the day I try the perfume.
I spray it all over my body
before I walk into my mother's arms.
Saturday, I sit dazed on the couch,
wondering what I will try next:
starched petticoats, dark chocolate,
a Brownie uniform from E-bay?
What will help her to remember?

How Mama Mailed a Letter

To mail a letter,
Mama licked the stamp
that would carry it far
from where she lived,
alone, Daddy gone,
and opened the front door
to stand there a minute
before she walked through,
her outfit perfect.
Down the road, left,
and up two blocks,
Mama walked, not to a mailbox
but to a bus stop
where she would wait,
her mail in the purse
strapped across her body.
She wore her watch
on her left wrist,
its Timex precision
exactly what she needed.
And then she rode downtown
to the corner of Main and Senate
to walk a block to Chick-fil-A,
where she ate one small piece of pie.
This she ate in a corner,
watching people come and go.
After this, she walked three blocks up
and two blocks down
to mail her letters and bills
at the main post office
before walking over to Laurel and Main,
three blocks from where her mother lived
when she worked at the YMCA,
to wait for another bus to get home.
Mama did this for years,

all the years she had walked on Main Street
intersecting in her memory
like a constellation of maps
even as dementia started to ride
with her downtown.
This is how she mailed a letter
until her children told her
it was time to stop taking buses
and she listened.

WHAT IT IS

It's your age.
I've been going a long time.
My falling, I fell this week.
I jumped up and I fell
and I had to push myself to my bed
and grabbed on it and got up.
My leg can hardly move.

George is going to take me to the doctor.
I just don't have sense enough to do it.
No food after 1 p.m.
Take me up to 15!

They called me and told me they had thirty things cheap.
We're gonna send it to you.
I ain't never seen it.
We're going out there tomorrow.

George is very smart.
He's more.
He did all the papers they wanted about her.
I said, "No, I don't remember."
I've fallen down so much.
I didn't heard the doctor.
He looked at me, head to foots.
My mind's been going out.

IV

let me miss my mother

At the Nursing Home

"I miss my mother," I tell Hattie,
shrugging guilt off my shoulders.
"You know, the way she was,
the way she used to be—
when she was healthy."
Not that we don't have a good time now.
And Hattie says, "She talks funny."
As if that sums it up,
as if that's the reason Audrey
lives in a nursing home.

It's all relative.
Audrey talks funny,
but she can tie her shoes.
When she wants to,
she can stand up and pour a cup of coffee
and sit down and cross her legs.
She can talk for hours,
and most everybody will listen,
even when she sounds like a robin.
Audrey can touch your shoulder
when you've had blood work,
and gesture at the bandage
and make a sad face.
She is allowed on the front porch
where she picks off all the dead flowers
and makes the others bloom.

It's all relative.
Which is why I can share my secret
with somebody who won't remember what I said
a day from now, but who will hold my hand,
and let me miss my mother,
my beautiful mother, who waves at Hattie and me now,
this precious moment,
from the other side of the room.

SATURDAY MORNING

Today I waved at Maggie with her sign
on the corner of Main and Cummings.
"Who's that?" my mother asked
as we drove by.
                    And I said, "Maggie."
I said, "Maggie is picketing for peace."

And my mother said, "That's nice."
Or something like that, waving too,
my sweet and senile mother
who danced with soldiers in 1944
and bought a beach towel in 1968
that said *Draft Beer Not Boys*
perhaps because it was on sale,
perhaps because she had three boys,
perhaps because she was legally blind.

One of the last things my mother told me,
when she could tell me things,
was what she thought of *this* war.

And so I waved at Maggie with her sign
on the corner of Main and Cummings
because she knows how to stand there
and stand there and stand there
with the patience of a child
and the simple optimism of mothers.

My Cheating Heart

Sometimes, if she's not all that very wet,
    and not a bit dirty down there when I peek,
        I check my mother out of her nursing home
without changing a thing—even if it means
    that I will have to spray the car with Lysol later
and spray extra Lysol on her wheelchair
    before we go into the coffee shop for coffee
        and her favorite cinnamon bun warmed over
            in the microwave for the two of us to share.
My mother likes to open the door to Java J's herself,
    wheeling through the tables and chairs she calls beautiful
    and past the mural of Venice painted on the wall.
Once we got to the cash register to order and a little girl stared,
    the glasses on her face reminding me of my mother's glasses
    that she wore from four to eighty-four and doesn't now.
It wasn't the wheelchair that caught her eye but my mother's kitten,
    her favorite stuffed toy that she traded for a moment with the girl,
    who handed her a small plastic purple horse with sparkling hair
that made my mother's eyes light up and made me forget she was wet,
    as wet as a toddler but not quite as wet as an 85-year-old can get
    after drinking watered-down coffee off and on since dawn.
The coffee shop we go to always smells like coffee beans,
    the rich aroma of my mother's favorite drink masking all else,
    the hot coffee as intoxicating as the cold wine she used to drink.

CLUES

A feather in her left hand,
tears in her eyes,
a laugh to right herself
as she falters.

Inside a folded bib,
a small white plush dog
now sepia with coffee stains.

I hold my mother's right hand.
We laugh together,
the feather foisted between us
like a thought lost
on a path through tears.

I tell her, "I will wash the dog."
I tell her, "The bird is not dead."

When she gives me the feather for keeps,
I put it in my pocket.
I wipe her tears.

Fate

Marge always wants to hold my hand,
Paula too—but she wants to caress it,
to run her fingers across my fingers
until she smiles and lets go, unlike Marge,
who never wants to let go and holds too tight.

With Paula, I feel like rosary beads.
With Marge, I am a life buoy
bobbing in rough water.

Bonita always reaches out when I walk past,
her hand poised to turn into a wave
if I don't reach right back and hold it.
Gerta rubs my hands if they are cold.
She would like to be my mother.

Audrey and I hold hands like sisters,
even though she is my mother
and I still feel like her daughter.
We are so close, the two of us,
she can read her future in my palm.

I can read my future too, in hers,
and in all these women's hands.

MISSING

My mother is missing a breast.
At Sunday dinner, no concentrated sugar allowed,
she pulls the fabric of her blouse and lets it fall
against her deflated chest.
   And then she points to the other one,
the one not even I, her daughter, suckled,
the one poised there like a teardrop.
I tell her they had to cut it off, that missing breast,
and smile and point to her plate.
"Here," I say. "You'll want to eat your turkey."
But she won't eat this white meat
pulled clean from the bone, soft and tender,
only yellow pudding sweetened artificially
and one slice of a bright orange yam.

She wants to be like everybody else, my mother.
She wants it all: two breasts, a real dessert,
a daughter whose white hair does not surprise her.
She wants to find the words to tell me she wants it all.
She wants to know who *they* are.

In the top drawer of a dresser she does not use,
my mother's prosthesis has a life of its own.
Neither jellyfish nor boob nor recyclable,
it lies in wait.
   One day, my mother will find her breast,
and she will want to play catch with it
or dress it up like a baby doll or eat it with a spoon.
"Here," I'll say. "You'll want to drink your milk."

ROLE PLAY WITH BEAR

I

Avuh, papuh—
frava frava freaqua,
kint owen.

Squook!

There's never never take put it anywhere.
Ha, ha.

Squook, squook, squook!

II

"What's he doing?" I ask,
pointing to her orange bear.

"He just waiting!" she answers,
looking at the bear in her lap,
dropping her "g" the way I do—
the way we both have always done.

Despite everything, my mother has not forgotten
how hard consonants can be
or how soft vowels can make everything,
from bears to bad news, bearable.

She just waiting too.

Emergency Room

Wisdom is the principal thing; therefore, get wisdom: and with all thy getting get understanding.—Proverbs 4

I do not think the doctor thinks I am intelligent.
I sense it in the way he talks to me, and pauses,
as if I will not understand what he is saying.
I think my comment about the CT scan classed me,
made me seem as if I have not read it all, and more,
as if studying Alzheimer's Disease has not been my life,
as if my mother's life has not been my life,
as if I am a total stranger to CT scans and brains.
We make conversation about the episode, though,
considering general observations and lab results
as he mentions all the tests he has performed.
I interrupt him once to tell him I am missing chemo
and wonder if I will die now, now that I am here,
holding my mother's hand in case she dies
instead of driving across town for treatment.
I can tell the doctor thinks I am worrying too much.
He tells me that I am not going to die.
My mother is not going to die either, not today.

Later, my mother will open her eyes and smile,
beatific in her innocence, happy to know I am there,
oblivious to emergency room and all its trappings.
Then the doctor will talk to *her* as if she understands
and I will realize that nothing is exactly as it seems,
that we are always where we need to be.
This doctor is not here for me but for my mother,
exactly where he needs to be at this moment in time:
explaining things clearly to me through my mother,
as if he never did doubt my intelligence,
as if I have the potential to understand.

The Other Night at Grace Healthcare & Rehabilitation

The other night,
I lay next to my mother
and let my hair fall against her face.

She giggled when it tickled her nose
and reached both hands out,
as if to hug me,
but she grabbed my hair instead—

gathering one pigtail in each fist—

and laughed some more,
as if she remembered exactly
what it means to mother.

BIRTHDAY

Mama put the daisy in her mouth,
and began to chew it whole,
so I held out my hand to her
in that universal gesture
of mother to child, or child to mother,
and she spit it out, petal by petal,
while I stared at her eyes,
instead of at the palm of my hand,
mesmerized by her confusion.

Earlier, I had taken a photo of it
as she held it, this white daisy,
thinking I might need a snapshot
to remember this afternoon.
It was my birthday, I was sharing,
a daisy and a piece of cake,
but the cake went untouched
the way *Happy Birthday* went unspoken
and I sang to myself in the car
as I drove home later, my hand still wet
with my mother's bitter spit.

V

wanting to find the words

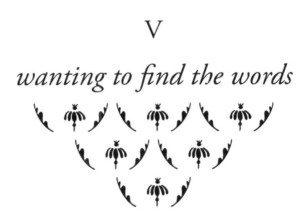

Second Childhood

I am not really a child,
even if I appear to be wearing diapers.
I am, in fact, wearing a diaper.
These sounds that come out of my mouth
are not coos and babbles, though,
or even words I know how to parrot,
so do not be fooled.
Everything I say makes sense.
I speak my own language,
the language of my own country,
like a native.
      I am a native speaker.
Before I came here to this place,
people questioned me,
asked me to repeat myself,
grinned at words they thought
I mispronounced.
Twice I was enrolled in elocution lessons!
Those teachers did not know Charleston,
did not know the way we all speak there,
thought we should speak like *them*.
Here nobody blinks an eye.
No matter what comes out of my mouth,
I get a look as if I said my first word
& not one that could be my last.
Here, the teachers feed me ice cream
& paint my fingernails.
My children bring me toys.
Somebody who is not my mother
tends to my diaper.

There is nothing wrong with toys.
More people should play with them.

I Am Still Here

I am still here.
My eyes are the keyhole
to a past we share.
Look into them,
and remember good times.
Even now, they glow
to light this unsteady path.
Let them help you
find your way.
Sometimes I may seem distant.
My ears remember your voice, though,
and music that I always loved
touches me,
the way your first word did.
If you ever worry you are losing me,
look into my eyes
and speak your first word,
the one only you and I know.
It will comfort us both.
And this nose,
it may not be able to smell
the foods it smells as well as it once did
or even let me eat them with zest,
but it is my nose.
It knows what pleases
and what offends,
and I appreciate every effort you make
to keep me smelling like
our favorite herbs and spices
instead of an institution.
I love the way you smell
and always welcome you into the room
even if I cringe sometimes
because my brain is confused
and thinks it doesn't recognize you—

but I know better.
I am more than my five senses.
I am here, right here, inside,
watching you, watching my brain,
watching what happens outside my window.
I taste the food you give me
and still give thanks.
I may not seem to have my senses,
but deep inside I do,
and I am watching you
the way a mother watches her children,
even as I am also watching myself,
wanting to find the words
to remind you that the soul
does not know the difference
between night and day
or young and old: it just is what it is,
the way your hand is what it is
when it touches mine
and lets me feel your pulse
because your pulse is my pulse.
I love you more now
than the day you were born,
even if it seems that I have moved
to a time before you were born.

ROOM

I have not left my bed for months,
not for days that feel like fleeting seconds,
my whole lifetime like a condensed book
between the sheets I lie in—
Valentine's Day, the ambulance came,
I went & came back here again—
but the orchid Felicia brought keeps blooming,
its colors as bright as that mobile that shimmers
when an aide touches it, lightly, gently, to make it tinkle,
the glass sound as colorful as a deep purple.

Sometimes an old man comes to sing to me,
playing his ukulele as if he thinks I like it,
but I do like him & his enthusiasm, his smile,
& so I smile at him & sometimes laugh.
He has the most beautiful white hair.
Sometimes young people clean my skin
or paint my fingernails or comb my hair
after my whole body is cleaned.
I never have to leave this bed for anything!
Propped on two pillows so I can see the window,
everything I need is tucked close by,
not out there where the sky meets a brick wall.
Even my meals come to me on angel wings,
& I am spoon-fed as if I am a child again
or a very old woman too weak to lift her arm
except to touch Felicia when she leans over me
to tend to one thing or the other.

SEVEN

I once read in *Reader's Digest*
how much the mind remembers—
seven, the magic number.
Seven words, seven ideas,
seven days in a bed, a week,
each like seven years at a time.
So much happens.
I try to hold onto seven.

Breakfast,
lunch,
supper,
bath,
sunshine,
sleep,
visits.

In between watching it all,
watching it all come and go in my room,
I watch the TV that is my doorway,
people coming & going past
before I can count to seven.

One,
two,
four,
seven,
seven.

Life's grand pageant is out there
with girls in crayon-colored scrubs,
& once a big white dog in overalls
that looked over at me and smiled.
If I could have walked out the door,
I would have followed that dog anywhere.

BALD FELICIA

My daughter is bald
underneath her scarf.
I can feel her bald head
when I pat her head.
I can see it, or not see it,
when she turns her back
to walk out that door
without a ponytail flopping.
She is trying to protect me
as I lie here in this bed,
but I remember chemo.
I know exactly what it means.

The two of us are the same,
two pieces of the same puzzle,
even if I chose to wear a wig.
When she leans down and hugs me—
her breast falling into the margins
where I once had another—
my one full breast fills in the gap
where her other breast is gone.
This is how we speak of cancer,
with our bodies instead of words.
Nothing comes between us.
It is as if we make each other
whole again—as whole as
a full head of hair or a healthy body.

Letting go of these last hugs
is teaching me how strong she is
and teaching my daughter
how to let go of me when I go.

THE TALK

For we brought nothing into this world, and it is certain we can carry nothing out.—Timothy 6:7

Everybody keeps having the talk with me,
first Felicia and then her friend Denise,
as if I need prodding to cross over.
My time will be my time when my time comes.
I want to leave this earth or body alone,
the way I came into it, alone, the way we all do,
& in a busy place like this house that takes planning.

A last meal will be nice, I think, dessert, coffee,
& an afternoon nap, no slipping away at night—
let me close my soul to rest my eyes
while the sun is shining in the window on my face
so I can wake up to an unclouded day—
no night in between the here and now—
that eternal day like the one I buried my son.

Denise described a heavenly shore.
Felicia listed everybody I will meet,
as if anybody will be there to greet me.
She knows me better than that.
Still, starting with Kitty-Boo, she named my cats,
every cat I ever knew and loved
(as if I might have forgotten all these cats)
along with Munny and my sisters and Daddy
& John Henry and John and everybody else
alleged to be there on the other side.
Felicia knows I never believed in another side.
It is certain we carry nothing out.
We are all just here now, all of us, together,
some alive, some dead, some visible, some invisible,
everybody & every cat & my last kitty,
my kitty, kitty, kitty.

My Last Favorite Bear

I never wanted a doll.
I know they like to give us dolls here.
I never wanted one.
I know the difference between a doll
and a baby, having birthed four.

Give me a plush animal any day,
like this oversized teddy bear,
as cuddly as a pillow.
Nobody will think I am stupid
if I talk to a toy bear.

Her dress is a blue plaid,
held on with buttons I like to unbutton
and button back and unbutton again.
White eyelet lace circles her skirt.
I can feel the stitches in the skirt,
stitches that remind me of my old Singer
and all the clothes I stitched with it.

One summer I sewed a bathing suit,
for me, a brilliant green floral suit
with a matching green skirt that swirled
like an ocean wave.
That was the year I bought blue plaid
for Felicia's dress and John Henry's shirt,
the two of them starting a new school.
We lived by the ocean then.

Pink checks and eyelet lace!
That is what I made for college dances,
Felicia's dances.

In between Easter dresses
and college dresses,

and a rabbit costume for Graeme,
I stitched miles of seams for me too,
my beautiful kaftans and dresses,
all as lovely as this bear's.

Look at my bear wearing pearls now,
as if she is as pretty as can be.

FEAR NOT

I can still read some words,
FEAR NOT among them
standing almost as tall as Jesus
on this piece of paper
I can hold in my own two hands.
A nice woman brought the words,
leaving them with a smile.

Jesus looks like John Henry.
He is enough to make me drop my fears
like a fork on this sanitary floor
where somebody mops daily—
John Henry, my son, who left this earth.
He was both afraid and not afraid.
And so young.
He died.

That is just the way it goes.
I do fear sometimes, true,
trapped here in a body that is not mine—
this old woman, who is she?
Unable to dress herself or pull a weed.
At least I know how to swim.
I do not know how to die.

Later, somebody will wash my hands,
wiping this newsprint off;
but, for now, I hold onto the paper
for dear life, my life,
my hands as gray as ash.

REGRETS

After Frank Sinatra and Edith Piaf

I had a few.
Too few to mention.
And then again,
I might as well mention
a few regrets.
I had a few.

If I could live my life over,
I would have been a farmer.

True, that is just the one regret.
Sometimes one regret
can feel a lot like
a few or even nothing.
Maybe I should say *rien de rien.*
I did it all my way.
I regret nothing.

But I had a few.

CODA

Dear Felicia,

I can see how green the leaves
are coming—
the tree outside my window
just gave birth to a bird.
One day soon,
a butterfly will fly by again,
but I will not know it is there.

Yesterday it rained,
diamonds on my windowpane,
ukulele music fluffing up my pillow.
A boy is sitting with me now.
He served my last meal and laughed
with me.

As happy as I am,
somebody gave me a pill
to calm me down.
I overheard her on the phone with you
explaining why,
telling you to get right over.
She thought I was thrashing,
fighting against the dying of the light,
but I was reaching out
to grab hold of my own mother—

and she was reaching back.

VI

stranger than fiction

LOVE IS STRANGE

Truth is stranger than fiction,
or at least a little more clichéd
when you come right down to it
and consider how the last word
my mother ever wrote—
in a steady, school-girlish hand—
was LOVE, even if she did copy it
letter by letter from a note I left
on an art pad with a sappy flower
drawn like something a kid would draw
for her mother, which is what I was,
I guess, a kid drawing for her mother,
shaping each petal into a balloon
in some off-kilter crayoned color
as if I was not over fifty
and my mother almost ninety.

The winged petals on my flower
make it look as if anything can fly.

THREADS

*Do not store up for yourselves treasures on earth, where
moths and vermin destroy*—Matthew 19

Unraveling the last hem my mother hemmed,
I finger the cotton thread as if I could follow it to her
instead of to the night she hemmed this coat,
her stitches steady but nothing like before—
nothing like stitches in the petticoat of my first dress.
I have this first Easter dress and little more.
If I had thought she would one day be gone,
I would have saved everything my mother ever stitched
instead of this store-bought coat with her last clumsy hem.
It was not a fair trade, a lifetime of dresses for this coat.

I think of my mother the last night in her home,
sitting in her chair by the last lamp she would own,
pulling white thread through gray wool to hem a coat
too large for her by all degrees, bought off the rack
by her son to keep her warm on her last trip, her trip to me.
For ten years, I have kept her coat in a chest,
pulling it out each autumn to finger the hem,
unable to let loose a coat too large for me to wear.
But now, today, I am letting go, forgetting the hem
and folding the coat as I think of how warm it will be
for somebody who would love to be warmer.
I know this is exactly what my mother wants,
so I hang the coat up to shake out the wrinkles,
then wind the thread I pulled from the hem, knots and all,
to tuck the talisman under a tuft of white hair
I keep in a porcelain bowl on the mantel
next to my favorite picture of my son.

FROSTED APRICOT

Mama was right.
The color is good on me—
though now, 16 years later,
it feels a little stale.
Why did I wait so long
to try the lipstick?
Why did I just look,
and shrug, and dismiss
another suggestion
to try to fix myself up?

She told me
I had so much more,
so much more to work with,
than she did.
She never believed.
She never believed
she was beautiful.
She thought I was,
or could be,
with just the right shade
of lipstick.

Today, cleaning my drawers,
I can wear the lipstick.
It looks good with my white hair.
I wish Mama could see me.
Or maybe she does.
Maybe even now,
even after death,
she knows she was right.

A Pansy for My Thoughts

Every February,
when she planted pansies
in the bed where daffodils bloomed,
Mama picked some
and wove them in my hair—

so that is how I walked to school
on my birthday until I lost count,
not so much a child of the Sixties
as my mother's child—

somebody closer to the earth
than to the sky above her
or the ocean across the bridge
or those people I'd see in their yards
looking longingly at stars.

Years later, one arrived in the mail,
passing from South Carolina to Texas,
a pansy folded in a card.

Now I plant them in February—
picking every color I find
at Kroger and K-Mart—
and I stare at them long and hard,
seeing my furrowed brow prophesied there,
something I did not see before,
when I wore pansies in my hair
and my mother remembered February.

BEAUFORT NATIONAL CEMETERY

It is hot when I arrive,
flowers from BI-LO in hand
to arrange in three containers
beneath broad oaks
where Spanish moss hangs,
shade in this summer's sun.
Daddy's flowers are white,
simple and quiet like him.
Mama's flowers are purple
because that is the color
she wore to marry Daddy.
My brother's flowers, yellow,
are cheerful against the lawn
that has blanketed him
for more than half my life.

I never know what to say
to my long-lost brother.
"Sorry" is what I say this time.
Sorry about the cancer,
sorry you died too young.
My father, a man of few words,
is happy for me to pause, silent.
It is easiest to talk to Mama.
Sometimes I kneel in the grass,
and other times I sit right down
as if I am going to have a picnic
although picnics are not allowed.
Today I tell her how lonely I am.
It is hard to live on this earth,
up here with the mockingbirds
and chiggers and people.
Even so, I try to fit into the world.
It is not my time to go.

After I visit all three graves
one more time, one more nod,
I run to a water sprinkler
that is watering the lawn and the dead
and dance like a child in the mist,
not quite ready to leave.

SILVER SERVICE

No amount of polish will restore the sheen,
the silver worn by soft hands and harsh detergent,
but the patches of gray and black among the silver
are as welcome as the silver threads among the gold hair
on my head as I grow older than my grandmother
who warmed the coffee pot with water from a well or tap.
One day I will serve myself a cup of coffee.
For now, I am content to watch a flower wilt
in the silver-plated vase I make of the coffee pot
with my grandmother's husband's initials engraved
as indelibly as my grandmother's stories are etched
on my tongue from inside my mother's mouth.

INHERITANCE

Phlox planted in the yard
returning every summer,
to remind me of the summer
I brought one plant here from home.

A model's coat with petunias
and my mother's name written on the collar,
a hand-me-down of a thrift-store bargain
my mother loved to wear, once.

One teddy bear dressed in a calico dress,
a diamond ring and a worn-out wedding band,
a teapot collection I never asked my mother
to explain to me when I could have asked.
The last lipstick she wore: Terra Cotta.

Three place settings of silver,
often tarnished but always sparkling
with memories of how I polished their silver
before my parents had to sell it,
all but two place settings for them
and one extra one for a visitor—
both of them always hopeful for a visitor.

Genes.
My son's beautiful blue eyes.
Resilience, almost as firm as my mother's.
An empty wallet with a check register
that is like a history of dementia
with the way words and numbers fall
across the years like a Rorschach blot
for me to interpret.
Sweatshirts embroidered *Audrey*,
enough to share with a cousin
as I spread my mother's wealth.
The way I look out of my eyes.

HINDSIGHT

After my mother is dead and buried,
I learn how her mother died—
a sad death in a mental asylum,
dead six days after being committed
by her own father when she was 41
for *emotional excitement*
due to undiagnosed psychosis.
This archaic diagnosis explains a lot.
It explains how my mother was cagey,
living alone past the time she should have,
only moving into a nursing home
when she was ready for 24-hour supervision
and had no choice in the matter.
It explains why she fought her fate.

It also explains how she stopped fighting,
as if she understood what the social worker said
when she told me she was weighing options
(nursing home versus another state hospital).
My mother could have lived her days out in either place,
her welfare already a public health concern
despite her family's interventions,
but she took a deep breath and went inside herself
to emerge a sweet and docile person,
the mother I remembered from early childhood,
a mother whose own inner child was strong.

I remember the exact moment I knew my mother
would do the best she could to be a good girl:
the moment I walked into her new home
and found her pushing a woman in a wheelchair.
"This is a big house," my mother said to me,
smiling a smile that came from finding family
after being lonely for so many years.

My mother never knew a stranger,
not on a city bus and not in a nursing home,
and this is how she thrived, vibrant, accepting,
a woman spoiled by three meals a day
and all the countless friends and family members
she could imagine or remember
in an institution that was nothing at all
like the one that swallowed up her mother.

CONTACT ERASED

How long do you hang on?
Until the cows come home,
or until the twelfth of never?

After I disconnected my mother's phone,
I kept her number in speed dial—
nestled next to an icon of a house,
a symbol I needed to hold onto.

But when I changed cell phones,
deleting numbers one by one,
I fingered this entry like the memory it was.

"Erase entry?" the phone asked me,
as articulate as a phone can be,
which is not all that much,
but more articulate than my mother was
with her alzheimerspeak.

I told it "yes" in cellphonespeak.
"Contact erased," the phone announced.
"Not really," I said aloud, talking back,
the way I would talk back to my mother
when she was in another room.
It's not as easy as all that.

BEDTIME STORY

Once upon a time, my mother once told me,
she took a history test:

Relate everything you have learned in this course
to the world situation today.

It was 1942.

I almost want to say that I would give anything
for some professor to find her blue book behind an oak bookcase
at the university where it could have fallen
and lain for decades after Audrey McClary took a pen and wrote,
long before a social worker came to her house
and asked her what year it was
and she couldn't say.

She never told me if she made an A or not, although she had to have.
A is, I think now, for artifact.

Underneath this story, there is another story determining its own destiny.
Remembering 1942 is not always an option,
but that doesn't mean it's gone.

Everything from Auschwitz to Audrey is there in somebody's memory.
You—we—just need to remember to pass it on.

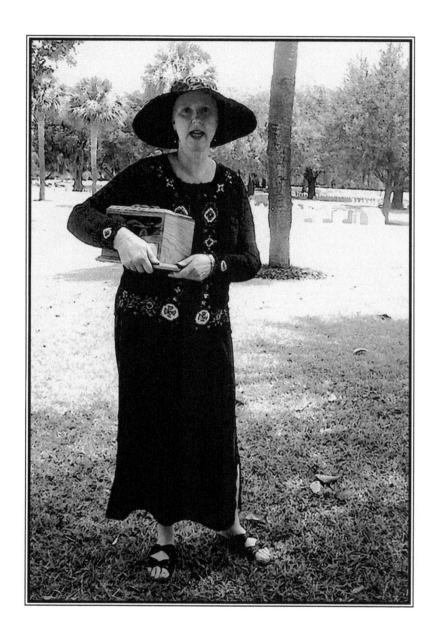

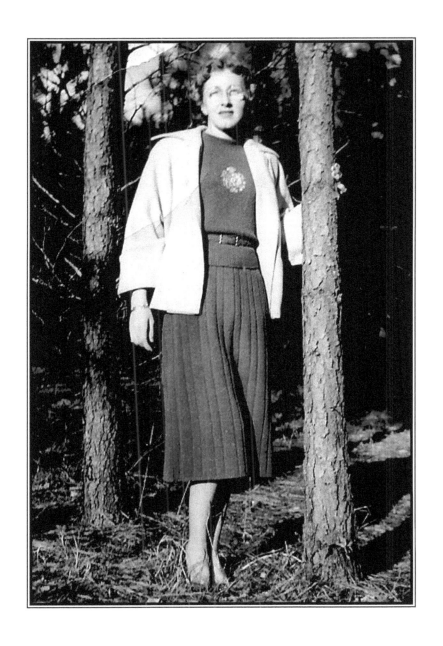

AFTERWORD

I hope this collection helps others to find ways to talk about dementia in new ways and see that those with dementia are not necessarily lost to us. I hope it starts conversations and inspires others to treasure the gifts of dementia that are embedded in the sad, challenging, and sometimes horrific times dementia inevitably brings. My main goal is to help us not to forget if we are able to remember. So many people will say to me about a loved one, "She does not know me! He has forgotten who I am!" That is not the point. The point is that we remember. We take over when our loved ones can no longer carry on in all ways. Journals, letters, diaries, video recordings—whatever helps us to remember who a loved one is will help this person through the years of living right there in the moment, just here now.

ACKNOWLEDGMENTS

When I first began imagining a book of poems with my mother's story, with her words interweaving with mine, I attended a Salzburg Seminar in Austria, "The Telling of Lives: Biography as a Mirror on Society," which helped this book to grow. Thanks thus are due to the Appalachian College Association and Emory & Henry College for sponsoring my attendance. Poems previously published in journals, anthologies, and a collection of my poems are acknowledged below, with grateful appreciation to the original publishers. Found poems were created from my mother's letters and notes I took during conversations. Identities of others in the nursing home were fictionalized. My images and family photos are used with permission, with author photo by Charles T. Mitchell.

Aileron: "Mama"

Bethlehem Writers Roundtable (the magazine of the Bethlehem Writers Group, LLC): "Frosted Apricot"

Bristol Cone: "Still Life with Cucumber"

Cleaning Up Glitter: "Intimation Ode"

Dead Mule School of Southern Literature: "A Pansy for My Thoughts," "At the S&S Cafeteria," "Saturday Morning," "Slop," "When is Summer?"

Hospital Drive: A Journal of Word and Image: "Role Play with Bear," "Contact Erased," "Fate"

Ink and Letters: "My Mother's Speech Impediment"

Low Explosions: Writings on the Body (edited by Casie Fedukovich with Steve Sparks for the Knoxville Writers' Guild, 2006): "Missing"

Motif. V2. Come What May: An Anthology of Writings about Chance (edited by Marianne Worthington for Motes Books, 2010): "Clues"

Out of Season: An Anthology of Work By and About Young People Who Died (edited by Paula Trachtman for Amagansett Press, 1992): "Mama"

Snapdragon: A Journal of Art and Healing: "Birthday," "Emergency Room"

Southern Women's Review: "The Other Night at Grace Healthcare & Rehabilitation"

Storms of the Inland Sea: Poems of Alzheimer's and Dementia Caregiving (edited by Margaret Stawowy and Jim Cokas for Shanti Arts Press, 2022): "My Cheating Heart"

Waltzing with Horses (written by Felicia Mitchell and published by Press 53, 2014): "At the S&S Cafeteria," "Missing," "The Other Night at Grace Healthcare & Rehabilitation," "Wateree Swamp"

About the Author

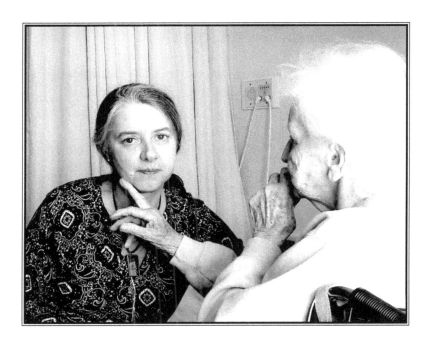

Felicia Mitchell was born in South Carolina and spent her childhood there and on the coast of North Carolina with her parents John A. and Audrey McClary Mitchell and three brothers. Following graduation from Booker T. Washington High School in Columbia, she received both BA and MA from the University of South Carolina. After completing a PhD at The University of Texas at Austin in 1987, she moved to rural southwestern Virginia, where she currently resides. Felicia taught English, including linguistics and creative writing, at Emory & Henry College for many years before retiring with emeritus status. Her scholarly work includes editing *Her Words. Diverse Voices in Contemporary Appalachian Women's Poetry.* Her poetry collections include *Waltzing with Horses* and a chapbook, *The Cleft of the Rock.* For ten years, she wrote a weekly column for *Washington County News* and, in recent years, she has blogged about experiences with cancer for *Cure Today.*

SELECTED BOOKS FROM WISING UP PRESS

FICTION

My Name Is Your Name & Other Stories
Kerry Langan

Germs of Truth
The Philosophical Transactions of Maria van Leeuwenhoek
Heather Tosteson

Not Native: Short Stories of Immigrant Life in an
In-Between World
Murali Kamma

Something Like Hope & Other Stories
William Cass

MEMOIR

Journeys with a Thousand Heroes: A Child Oncologist's Story
John Graham-Pole

Keys to the Kingdom: Reflections on Music and the Mind
Kathleen L. Housley

Last Flight Out: Living, Loving & Leaving
Phyllis A. Langton

POETRY

Source Notes: Seventh Decade
Heather Tosteson

A Hymn that Meanders
Maria Nazos

Epiphanies
Kathleen L. Housley

A Little Book of Living Through the Day
David Breeden

PLAYS

Trucker Rhapsody & Other Plays
Toni Press-Coffman

WISING UP ANTHOLOGIES

ILLNESS & GRACE: TERROR & TRANSFORMATION

FAMILIES: *The Frontline of Pluralism*

LOVE AFTER 70

DOUBLE LIVES, REINVENTION & THOSE WE LEAVE BEHIND

VIEW FROM THE BED: VIEW FROM THE BEDSIDE

SHIFTING BALANCE SHEETS:
Women's Stories of Naturalized Citizenship & Cultural Attachment

COMPLEX ALLEGIANCES:
Constellations of Immigration, Citizenship & Belonging

DARING TO REPAIR: *What Is It, Who Does It & Why?*

CONNECTED: *What Remains As We All Change*

CREATIVITY & CONSTRAINT

SIBLINGS: *Our First Macrocosm*

THE KINDNESS OF STRANGERS

SURPRISED BY JOY

CROSSING CLASS: *The Invisible Wall*

RE-CREATING OUR COMMON CHORD

GOODNESS

FLIP SIDES:
*Truth, Fair Play & Other Myths We Choose to Live By:
Spot Cleaning Our Dirty Laundry*

ADULT CHILDREN:
Being One, Having One & What Goes In-Between

Lightning Source UK Ltd.
Milton Keynes UK
UKHW010754270922
409514UK00001B/145